THE PROFESSIONAL POSTURE PROGRAM

Upgrade Your Upright

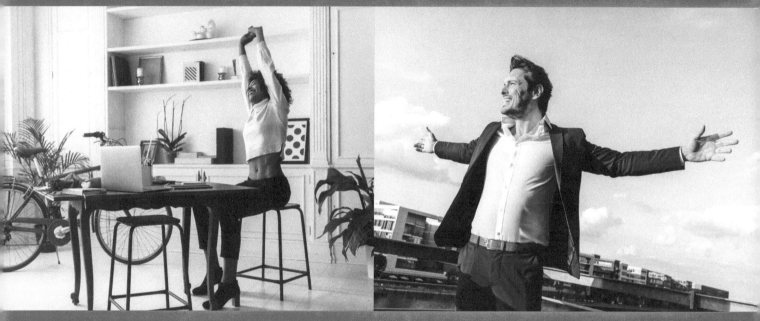

Work-Friendly Yoga Exercises
To Improve Posture, Health and Confidence

Do At Your Desk
At the Office Or At Home

Less than 15 minutes a day

Walid Hafez, MD   **Zachary Hafez, MD**

Amina Hafez, certified yoga instructor

The Desk Manual for Every Desk

THE PROFESSIONAL POSTURE PROGRAM

WORK-FRIENDLY YOGA EXERCISES
TO IMPROVE POSTURE, HEALTH AND CONFIDENCE

Do At Your Desk
At the Office or At Home

WALID HAFEZ, MD, ZACHARY HAFEZ, MD,

AND

AMINA HAFEZ, CERTIFIED YOGA INSTRUCTOR

The Professional Posture Program

To order additional copies of this book, contact:
Xlibris
844-714-8691
www.Xlibris.com
Orders@Xlibris.com

The website and references contained within this book are intended to serve as resources with no guarantee expressed or implied as to the accuracy of their content.

ISBN: 978-1-9845-8701-5 (sc)
ISBN: 978-1-9845-8702-2 (hc)
ISBN: 978-1-9845-8700-8 (e)

Library of Congress Control Number: 2020912963

Print information available on the last page

Rev. date: 08/31/2020

CONTENTS

Introduction ix

Chapter 1 Advantages of Having Good Posture 3

Chapter 2 What Is Posture? 9

Chapter 3 How Can I Get and Maintain Good Posture? 19

Chapter 4 The Exercises: Daily Workday Sequence 29

Chapter 5 Bonus Exercises 43

Chapter 6 Common Questions about the Exercises (with Answers) 55

Appendix Reference Sheets to Post at Your Desk 57

Acknowledgments 77

About the Authors 78

FOR SHARON

INTRODUCTION

Our health is the net result of our choices and genetics, as well as unforeseen circumstances. We do have substantial control over our behavior and the positive decisions we make. Our choices—with respect to exercise, stress reduction, diet and sleep—provide us with a continuum of opportunities to improve the quality of our lives. To be successful in steadfastly making positive choices, we need a disciplined approach that is doable. Selecting and committing to a practical program will help us to achieve our goals.

Our exercise goals should include exercising for good posture. Proper posture is one of the most important factors in preventing long-term, chronic neck and back pain, which are among the most frequent causes for which people seek medical care, either from a primary doctor or in an emergency setting. In addition to reducing neck and back pain, proper posture promotes improved lung expansion, which improves blood oxygenation and helps reduce fatigue and improve cognition and energy levels.

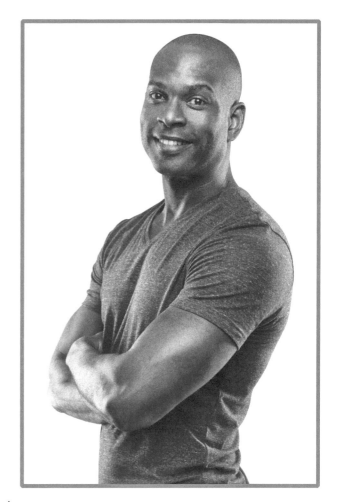

The program offered in this book is practicable. It can be comfortably and easily implemented one or more times a day—during the workday, at one's desk—with noticeable benefits within a few weeks. The daily recommended exercises are in keeping with sound physiological, medical and physical principles applied in rehabilitation and health promotion. Once you start this program, your body and mind will request you to keep applying yourself to a disciplined, planned exercise and mindfulness activity.

This program is worth your time, effort, and immediate and long-term health.

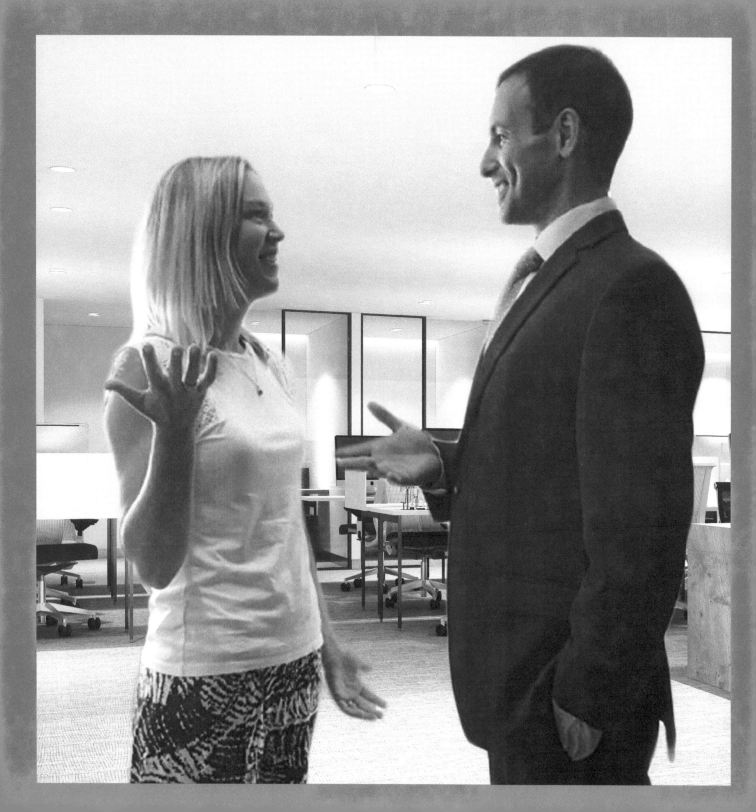

CHAPTER 1:
ADVANTAGES OF HAVING GOOD POSTURE

Having good posture has several advantages for working professionals. It helps to keep your physical body functioning optimally so you can perform your best. It helps support your productivity and confidence. It also enhances your professional image.

Keeps you physically healthy. Having good posture will help keep you physically healthy by reducing your likelihood of headaches and neck, shoulder, back and knee pain. You will also burn more calories since having good posture

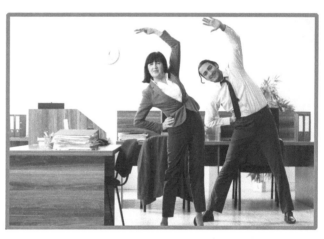
Exercise for good posture to stay physically healthy.

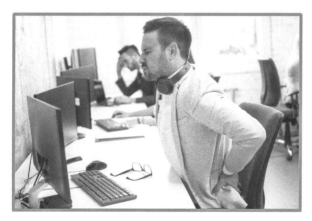
Bad posture can lead to numerous negative health consequences, including back pain.

requires you to work your core muscles. With good posture, your quality of breath will improve as your body takes in more oxygen, which helps improve your immunity and the effectiveness of your nervous system and other organs.[1]

1 Janet T. Hein, "Posture: Align yourself for good health," *Mayo Clinic*, December 14, 2016, https://www.mayoclinic.org/healthy-lifestyle/adult-health/in-depth/posture-align-yourself-for-good-health/art-20269950/

On the other hand, bad posture can lead to negative health consequences, causing headaches and migraines, neck and back pain, muscle and joint tension, fatigue, poor circulation and lung compression. It can make you more susceptible to injury. According to the Chartered Society of Physiotherapy, "Posture ranks right up at the top of the list when you are talking about good health. It is as important as eating right, exercising, getting a good night's sleep and avoiding potentially harmful substances like alcohol, drugs and tobacco."[2] As a working professional, your health is an important concern not only to you, but also to your employer, business partners and investors. Therefore, it pays to invest your time in performing daily exercises during the workday to support good posture.

Enhances your productivity and emotional well-being. Good posture helps keep your mental fitness sharp so you can continue to sustain the high-pressure demands of your job. Studies show that having good posture makes you remarkably more productive—it increases your energy, improves concentration and alertness, and helps build resilience to stress.[3] However, having poor posture can make you

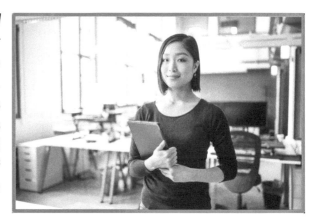

Good posture makes you more productive.

---

2 James Crossley. *Personal Training: Theory and Practice* (Routledge, 2013).

3 Shwetha Nair, Mark Sagar, John Sollers, Nathan Consedine, Elizabeth Broadbent, "Do Slumped and Upright Postures Affect Stress Responses? A Randomized Trial." Health Psychology: Official Journal of the Division of Health Psychology, American Psychological Association, September 2014, 34(6), 632–641, https://doi.org/10.1037/hea0000146. See also Erik Peper, Annette Booiman, I-Mei Lin, Richard Harvey. "Increase Strength and Mood with Posture," Beweegreden 12. 14–17. 10.5298/1081-5937-44.2.04 (2016), https://www.researchgate.net/publication/303540780_Increase_Strength_and_Mood_with_Posture. Erik Peper and I-Mei Lin. "Increase or Decrease Depression: How Body Postures Influence Your Energy Level," Biofeedback: Fall 2012, Vol. 40, No. 3, pp. 125–130, https://doi.org/10.5298/1081-5937-40.3.01

feel drained, lethargic and unfocused, which decreases your productivity.[4] There is real value to your career in investing in your posture.

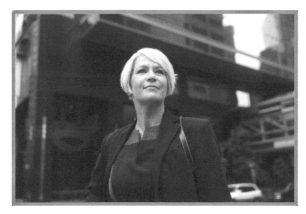
Good posture can make you feel more confident and optimistic.

Good posture can also promote confidence and other leadership qualities. Research shows that people with good upright posture are likely to feel more confident, assertive, dominant and proactive, have increased self-esteem, and be more optimistic and more comfortable taking risks.[5] One reason for this is the increased level of testosterone and decreased level of stress

hormones that your body produces as a result of holding an upright, expansive posture. With good posture, you will not have to fake it until you make it. Having good posture will help you

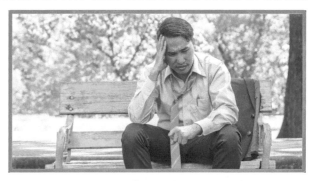
Poor posture can foster depression, feelings of helplessness and higher stress.

4 Erik Peper, Annette Booiman, I-Mei Lin, Richard Harvey, "Increase Strength and Mood with Posture," Beweegreden 12 (2016), 14-17, 10.5298/1081-5937-44.2.04, https://www.researchgate.net/publication/303540780_Increase_Strength_and_Mood_with_Posture. See also Erik Peper and I-Mei Lin, "Increase or Decrease Depression: How Body Postures Influence Your Energy Level," Biofeedback: Fall 2012, Vol. 40, No. 3, pp. 125-130, https://doi.org/10.5298/1081-5937-40.3.01.
5 Dana R. Carney, Amy J.C. Cuddy, Andy J. Yap, "Power Posing: Brief Nonverbal Displays Affect Neuroendocrine Levels and Risk Tolerance," Psychological Science, 2010, faculty.haas.berkeley.edu. See also Ohio State University, "Body Posture Affects Confidence in Your Own Thoughts, Study Finds," ScienceDaily, 5 October 2009, www.sciencedaily.com/releases/2009/10/091005111627.htm; University of Southern California, "Your Mother Was Right: Good Posture Makes You Tougher," ScienceDaily, 13 July 2011, www.sciencedaily.com/releases/2011/07/110712133337.htm; V.E. Wilson, E. Peper, "The Effects of Upright and Slumped Postures on the Recall of Positive and Negative Thoughts," Appl Psychophysiol Biofeedback 29, 189–195 (2004), https://doi.org/10.1023/B:APBI.0000039057.32963.34.

internalize confidence, which in turn will better enable you to project a powerful, professional image more convincingly.

Conversely, studies show that having poor posture can foster depression, feelings of helplessness and higher stress.[6] Professionals and aspiring professionals experiencing these types of feelings will have difficulty motivating and inspiring others. Performing daily exercises to achieve and maintain good posture will give you an advantage in generating enthusiasm and passion to influence others more effectively.

Improves your professional image. Good posture enhances your professional image. Like it or not, your effectiveness as a leader and communicator is impacted by the impressions you make in a meeting. While there is no magic formula for commanding a room or projecting a powerful appearance, having good posture is an important component of executive presence.

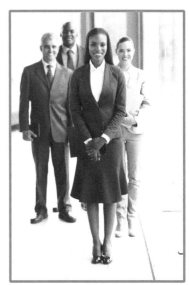

Good posture enhances your professional image.

Having upright, expansive posture reflects high power and status and makes you come across to others as more authoritative and dominant.[7] This reinforces your professional look, conveying strength and confidence, which helps further a positive perception of your communication and leadership abilities. On the other hand, having a slumped posture broadcasts weakness and submissiveness—not an image that will help you influence or attract others to your vision or cause. Good posture also helps with your visual appearance, making you look taller, slimmer and healthier, which bolsters a more attractive, successful image and makes a more powerful first impression.

6 Erik Peper, Annette Booiman, I-Mei Lin, Richard Harvey, "Increase Strength and Mood with Posture," Beweegreden, 2016, 12. 14-17. 10.5298/1081-5937-44.2.04, https://www.researchgate.net/publication/303540780_Increase_Strength_and_Mood_with_Posture. See also JZ Canales, TA Cordas, JT Fiquer, AF Cavalcante, RA Moreno, "Posture and Body Image in Individuals with Major Depressive Disorder: A Controlled Study," Brazilian Journal of Psychiatry, 2010 Dec.; 32(4):375-80, https://doi.org/10.1590/S1516-44462010000400010.
7 Li Huang, Adam Galinsky, Deborah Gruenfeld, and Lucia Guillory, "Powerful Postures Versus Powerful Roles," Psychological Science (2011), 22. 95-102, https://doi.org/10.1177/0956797610391912.

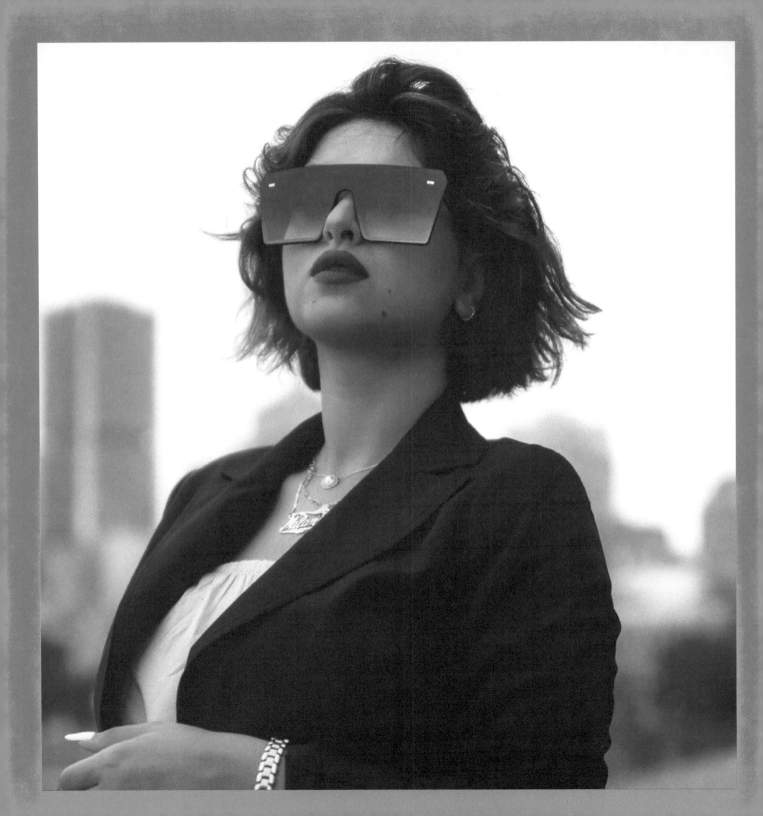

CHAPTER 2:
WHAT IS POSTURE?

Simply put, posture is your body's alignment to the effects of gravity at any given point in time. It is the way you hold your body while sitting, standing, lying down or moving. During a typical day, you take on many different postures depending upon what you are doing. You cannot live your life in one posture.

Good posture places your body in the best alignment for it to absorb external stress, minimizing wear and tear on your muscles, ligaments, joints and bones. Key to good posture is your back and the position of your spine. A healthy spine is a smooth S-shape with three natural curves. The cervical spine (neck area) has a concave, inward arch, or lordosis. The thoracic spine (upper back) has a convex, outward arch, or kyphosis. The lumbar spine (lower back), like the cervical spine, also has a lordotic curve. The spine terminates at the sacrum and coccyx. The lumbosacral junction, which consists of the L5 vertebral body articulating with the first sacral vertebral body, affects the mobility of the spine.

Good posture means maintaining the spine's natural curves. Your entire body impacts your posture, from the position of your head to your feet. Any increase or flattening of your spine's curves will create a postural imbalance.

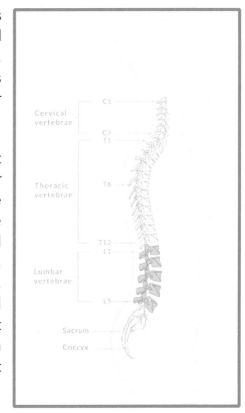

An example of a healthy spine, a smooth S-shape with three natural curves – cervical, thoracic and lumbar.

You maintain these curves by aligning:

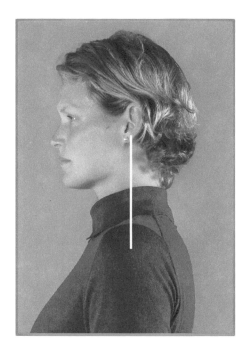

- your **ears** over your **shoulders**,

- your **shoulders** over your **hips**,

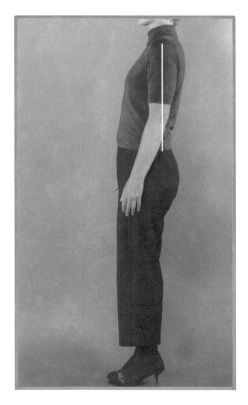

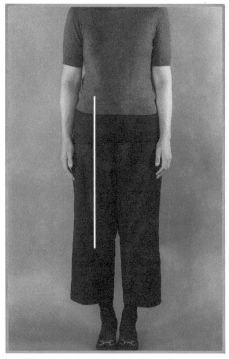

- your **hips** over your **knees**, and

- your **knees** over your **ankles**.

Good Posture – Standing

To stand with good posture:

- Stand with feet hip-width apart, weight divided equally between your feet, more toward the balls of your feet.

- Slightly bend your knees.

- Keep your hips aligned over your knees by flexing your glutes, tucking your pelvis under slightly.

- Pull your abdomen in.

- Lengthen your spine.

- Roll your shoulders back and down.

- Keep your ears back over your shoulders.

- Keep your chin level, parallel to the ground.

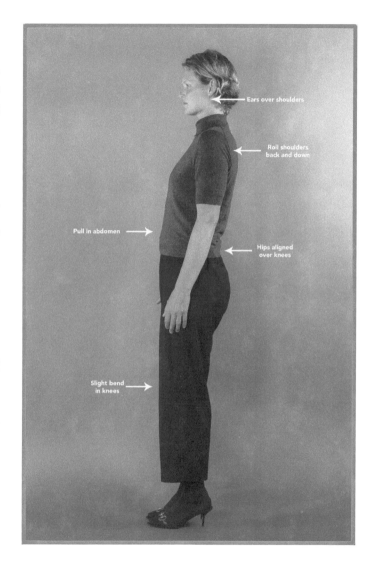

You can also check your posture by standing with your back against a wall, with the back of your head, shoulders and glutes touching the wall, and your heels approximately two inches away from the wall.

Watch out that these common bad postural habits do not develop

Head position. Watch that your head does not jut forward (where your ears are in front of your shoulders) or to one side.

Shoulders. Do not round or hunch your shoulders forward.

Back. Do not excessively round your upper back.

Hips. Be mindful that your pelvis does not tilt forward. Tuck glutes in.

Knees. Do not lock your knees.

Feet. No subway or bus stop stance. Do not put more weight on one foot.

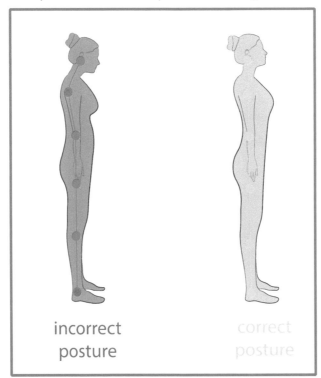

Examples of incorrect and correct
standing postural alignment.

Good Posture – Seated

Having a good chair that properly supports your body is key to sitting with good posture. To sit with good posture:

- Sit all the way back in the chair so that your glutes touch the chairback.

- Place your feet flat on the floor or on a footrest.

- Your knees should be directly above your ankles and in line with your hips so that your thighs are parallel to the floor (and your shins are at right angles to your thighs).

- Keep your elbows close to your torso. **Bend your elbows no less than 90 degrees and no more than 120 degrees.**

- Relax your shoulders.

- Lengthen your spine and neck.

- Keep your ears directly over your shoulders.

- Stretch the top of your head toward the ceiling and tuck your chin in slightly.

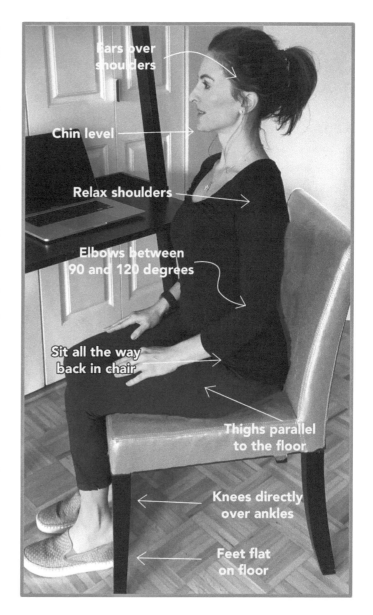

Ears over shoulders

Chin level

Relax shoulders

Elbows between 90 and 120 degrees

Sit all the way back in chair

Thighs parallel to the floor

Knees directly over ankles

Feet flat on floor

Watch out that these common bad postural habits do not develop

Head position. Watch that your head does not jut forward.

Shoulders. Do not round or hunch your shoulders forward.

Back. Do not sit with hyperlordosis of the lower back or hyperkyphosis of the upper back.

Torso. If sitting in a swivel chair, do not twist.

Legs. Do not cross your legs for extended periods.

Hips and knees. Make sure that your knees are in line with your hips.

Feet. Keep your feet flat on the floor.

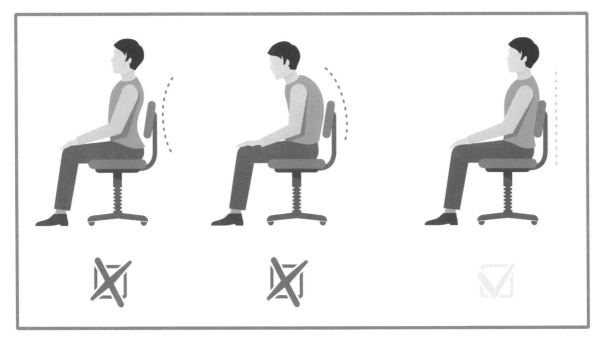

Image on left demonstrates a hyperlordotic lumbar spine. Middle image illustrates a hyperkyphotic thoracic spine. Image on right illustrates proper spinal alignment.

Desk Posture

When seated or standing at a desk in front of a computer, there are a few additional positions to which you need to pay attention:

- **Monitor.** Your eyes should be level with the top of the monitor, so that your chin is parallel to the floor when you look at the screen. If you are working with two monitors side by side equally, arrange your position so that you are looking in the middle of both screens. If you use one monitor more frequently, place this monitor directly in front of you.

- **Keyboard and Mouse.** Make sure your keyboard and mouse are positioned so that your forearms are parallel to the floor and your elbows bend **no less than 90 degrees** and **no more than 120 degrees**.

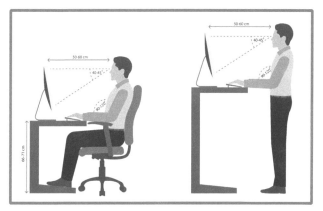

Examples of proper desk and technology set-ups for seated and standing desk positions. Important to keep eyes level with the top of the monitor and to keep elbows bent no less than 90 degrees and no more than 120 degrees.

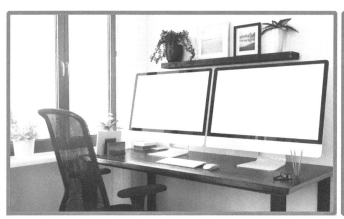

Dual monitors.

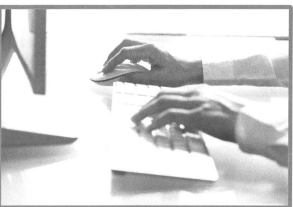

Forearms parallel to the floor.

- **Desk**. If sitting, your legs should have sufficient space under your desk. Create optimal space for your knees, thighs and feet by

  - adjusting your chair height,
  - raising the desk (e.g., using a desk lifter), and/or
  - using a footrest.

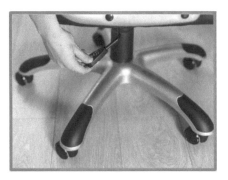

Adjustable chair.

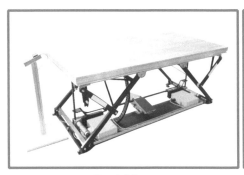

Desk lifter.

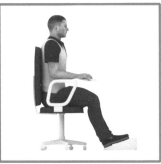

Footrest.

- **Headset.** Use a headset or speakerphone to avoid holding your phone and cranking your neck.

- **Document Holder.** Use a document holder to hold your documents upright while you read them in order to avoid looking down for extended periods of time.

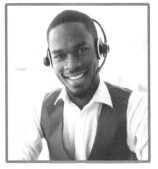

Headset.

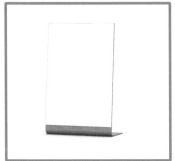

Document stand.

Why am I at risk for bad posture?

Anyone who sits at a desk or looks at a computer, smartphone, tablet or down at reading materials is at risk for acquiring bad posture. What happens when this occurs for extended periods of time is that your body becomes fatigued, and your shoulders start to round forward. As you stare at your computer, you might notice that you are leaning forward to read the screen, or even extending out your neck. The same thing happens when we stare at our smartphone or tablet. Our bodies begin to hunch toward the device. In addition, if we sit for extended periods of time, our hip flexors and hamstrings begin to tighten. As Aristotle, the ancient Greek philosopher, once stated, "We are what we repeatedly do." Holding your body in these positions every day for extended periods of time will cause your body to get good at these postural misalignments, and you will inevitably develop postural imbalance.

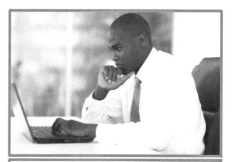

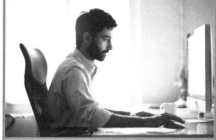

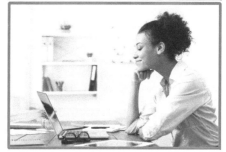

Persons at high risk for developing postural imbalance (hyperkyphotic thoracic spine, rounding forward of the shoulders and extension of the neck)

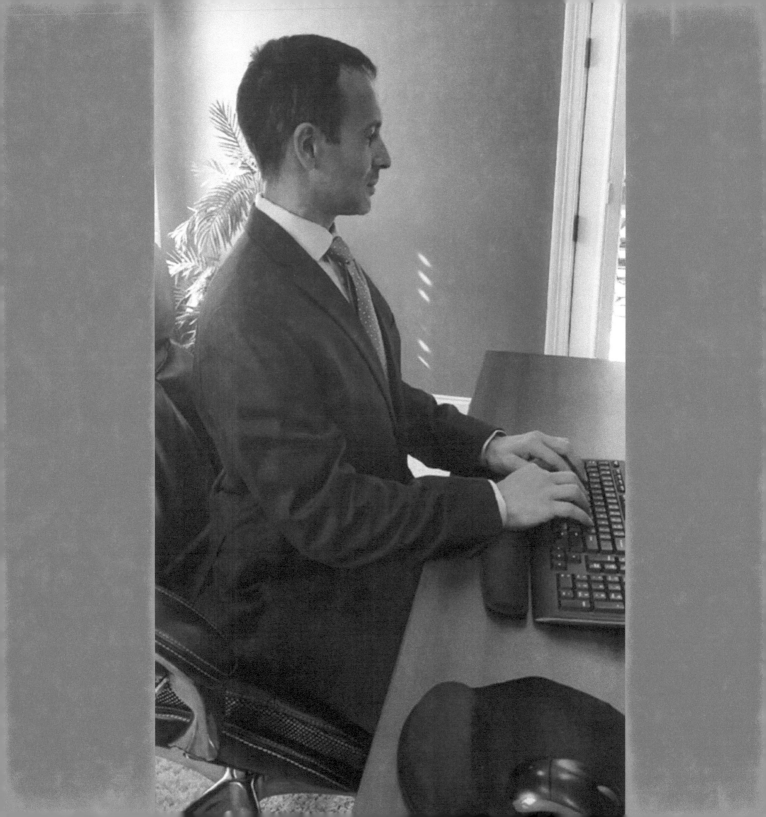

CHAPTER 3:

HOW CAN I GET AND MAINTAIN GOOD POSTURE?

To get and keep good posture, you must be vigilant about working on your alignment—it needs to be a habit. In today's technological society, you must fight for good posture every day by performing targeted exercises that counteract looking down (e.g., at your technology device) and sitting for extended periods. A hunched position is a result of having tight neck, chest and shoulder muscles and weak upper back muscles. Lower back and knee pain results from having tight hip flexors and hamstrings. Therefore, to get and maintain good posture, you must *daily* (1) stretch the muscles in your neck, chest and shoulders, (2) strengthen the muscles in your back, (3) stretch your hip flexors and hamstrings, and (4) become increasingly present and aware of your postural alignment.

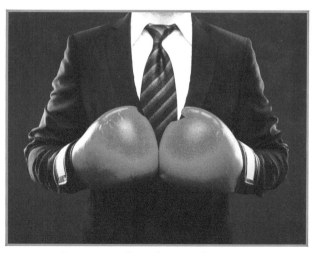

Commit to fight for good posture.

Ergonomics and the Importance of Your Desk Set-Up

Awareness of your postural alignment includes paying attention to proper ergonomics and your desk set-up. Your desk, chair, monitor, keyboard and mouse should all be carefully adjusted to accommodate good posture (see discussion in Chapter 2). Your chair should have adequate support for the lower back, which helps your back muscles relax as you sit and work. If working at a seated desk position, you should try to walk around or do some desk exercises every 30 minutes.

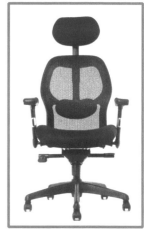

Ergonomic
office chair.

Many companies provide ergonomics assessments for your desk set-up when you are at the office. However, you should also make sure that your home workstation is ergonomically correct. If you use a laptop computer in your home office, you should evaluate whether you need to purchase a laptop stand in order to raise the screen to your eye level so that you avoid looking down, which causes stress on your neck, shoulders and back. You should also assess whether you need a second keyboard and an ergonomic keyboard tray so that you can maintain your wrists level and bend your elbows no less than 90 degrees and no more than 120 degrees when you type.

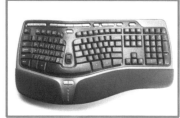

Ergonomic keyboard.

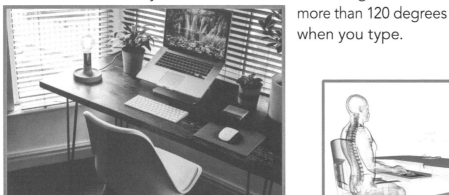

Ergonomic home office. Laptop is raised on a stand so that the screen is positioned at eye level. A second keyboard allows elbows to be bent between 90 and 120 degrees with forearms parallel to the floor.

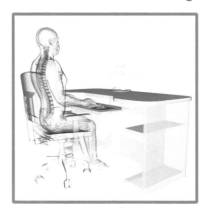

Ergonomic keyboard tray.

Posture Correctors Can Supplement (But Not Replace) Daily Exercises

Today, there are many posture corrector devices that can help you find your best posture and make you more aware of your posture when you are sitting and standing. Generally, these devices are best used in small doses so that your muscles do not become dependent on them and weaken. While these devices can be helpful to increase your awareness of your posture, they must be used in tandem with a daily stretching and strengthening program. In other words, even if you use a posture corrector to assist you, it is not a replacement for your daily posture exercises.

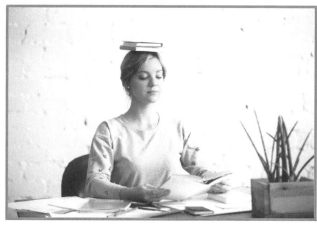
Traditional posture corrector.

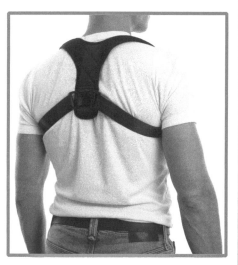
Backbrace posture corrector.

What are examples of posture correctors? Posture correctors come in all shapes and sizes, including:

- Backbraces with options that can be worn over or under clothing (e.g., Evoke Pro A300 Posture Corrector)

- Device that attaches to your back and vibrates when you start to slouch (e.g., Upright GO Posture Trainer and Corrector)

- Posture belt that allows you to sit ergonomically in any chair (e.g., BetterBack)

- Posture corrector bras (e.g., Leonisa Perfect Everyday Posture Corrector Underwire Cami Sports Bra with Back Support)

Postural Pitfalls and Quick Fixes

Below are some common postural pitfalls for which you should practice to develop heightened awareness, as well as some quick fixes for you to implement should you catch yourself indulging in any of these pitfalls.

Head and Neck

Common Pitfalls. The head is an extension of the spine. Keeping your ears directly above your shoulders will keep your head and neck in proper postural alignment. However, if you are prone to rolling your shoulders forward and rounding your upper back (a hyperkyphotic posture of the thoracic spine), this will cause your head to push forward of the shoulders and your chin to jut out, causing forward-head posture (also called text-neck or tech-neck). For every inch that your head pushes forward away from proper postural alignment, your head's weight-load increases by 10 pounds on the rest of your body to support your head. This increased postural stress places greater strain on your neck, shoulders and upper back. Not surprisingly, this can lead to headaches and neck, shoulder and back pain.

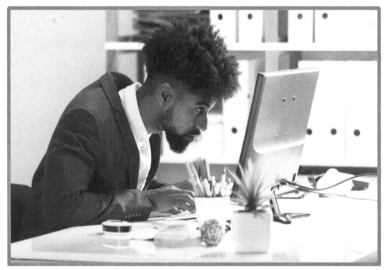

Forward head posture, a.k.a. tech-neck or text-next.

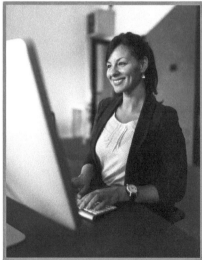

Proper head and shoulder alignment.

Quick Fix Solutions. Be vigilant that your ears stay over your shoulders.

Quick Fix #1 –*Lift Ribcage*. To foster this alignment, take the rounding out of your upper back by rolling your shoulders back and down and lifting your ribcage. Imagine that you have headlights on your collar bones and upper ribs and that you are beaming the headlights out and up. This will cause your chest to lift, which will draw your head back and reduce the rounding in your back.

Quick Fix #2 – *Stretch the Back of Your Neck*. Keep the muscles in the base of your head and the back of your neck limber by stretching them. Do this by performing chin tuck holds (see Chin Tuck exercise below).

Chest and Shoulders

Common Pitfalls. With good postural alignment, your shoulders should be directly above your hips. However, any activity that causes you to look forward and down for prolonged periods of time (e.g., texting, typing on a laptop, surfing on a tablet) can encourage your shoulders to move forward, in front of your hips. This position can cause increased stress on the shoulder joints, causing pain in the neck and upper back.

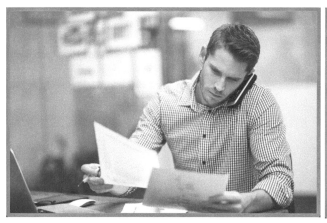

Shoulders rounded too far forward, not in line with hips. Also poor neck posture (should use headphones or a headset).

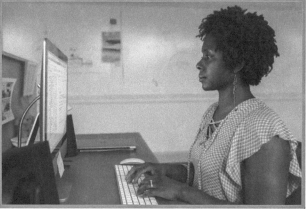

Proper alignment of shoulders directly over hips.

Quick Fix Solutions. Keep your shoulders aligned directly over your hips.

Quick Fix #1 – *Roll Shoulders Back.* Rolling your shoulders back and drawing your shoulder blades in and down your back will bring your shoulders back to be more in line with your hips.

Quick Fix #2 – *Lift the Chest.* Lengthen your chest by lifting the top of your sternum toward the ceiling. Broaden your chest across the collar bones. This will cause your chest to lift, which will also draw your shoulders back.

Back

Common Pitfalls. Hunching or slumping forward for extended periods of time can cause your upper and mid back muscles to weaken and your chest muscles to tighten. As a result, your upper back and thoracic spine may become characterized by increased kyphosis or excessive rounding. To achieve proper alignment of the spine, it is necessary to strengthen the back muscles and increase flexibility in the chest.

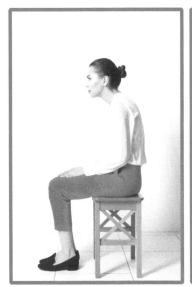 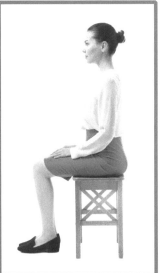

Increased kyphosis
(excessive rounding of
the thoracic spine).

Proper spinal alignment.

Quick Fix Solutions. Engage your back and core muscles to help support your shoulder alignment directly over your hips.

Quick Fix #1 – *Engage Your Back and Core Muscles.* As you roll your shoulders back, draw your shoulder blades in and down your back, squeezing them together as if there were a pencil in between them (see Shoulder Blade Squeeze exercise below). You should start to feel your trapezius and rhomboid muscles working. Engage your core muscles by pulling your abdomen in while lifting your ribcage.

Quick Fix #2 – *Stretch Your Chest.* Keep the muscles in your chest limber by stretching them. Do this by performing a chest/pectoralis stretch (see Chest Stretch at Wall or Doorframe exercise below).

Hips

Common Pitfalls. When you sit for long periods of time, your hip flexors are in a constant state of flexion. Over time, this causes these muscles to shorten and become tight. Tight hip flexors will pull your pelvis down and forward, which compresses your lower back and causes your tailbone to lift. An anterior pelvic tilt and hyperlordotic lumbar curve, or swayback, will soon develop, which means that your rear will be sticking out. This creates a postural imbalance as your pelvis is forward of your knees and no longer in alignment with the spine, knees and ankles.

In addition, sitting for long periods of time causes tight hamstrings. Tight hamstrings will pull on your lumbar spine and cause low back pain.

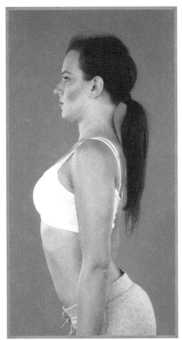
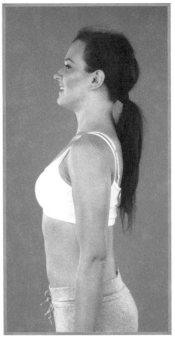

Anterior pelvic tilt and hyperlordotic lumbar curve, or swayback.

Proper pelvic alignment.

Quick Fix Solutions. Keep flexibility in your hip flexors and hamstrings.

Quick Fix #1 – *Stretch Your Hip Flexors.* For proper standing posture, it is important to keep your hips in alignment with your shoulders above, and your knees and ankles below. Perform hip flexor stretches (see Seated Lunge exercise below).

Quick Fix #2 – *Squeeze Your Glutes While Pulling Your Abdomen In.* When you squeeze your glutes, the pelvis rotates back under the body to a neutral position. Pulling your abdomen in while squeezing your glutes causes your navel to move in toward the spine, your chest to come forward, your shoulders to go back, and your neck and head to lengthen upward.

Quick Fix #3 – *Stretch Your Hamstrings.* Perform hamstring stretches to keep your hamstrings flexible, preventing them from pulling on your low back (see Hamstring Stretch exercise below).

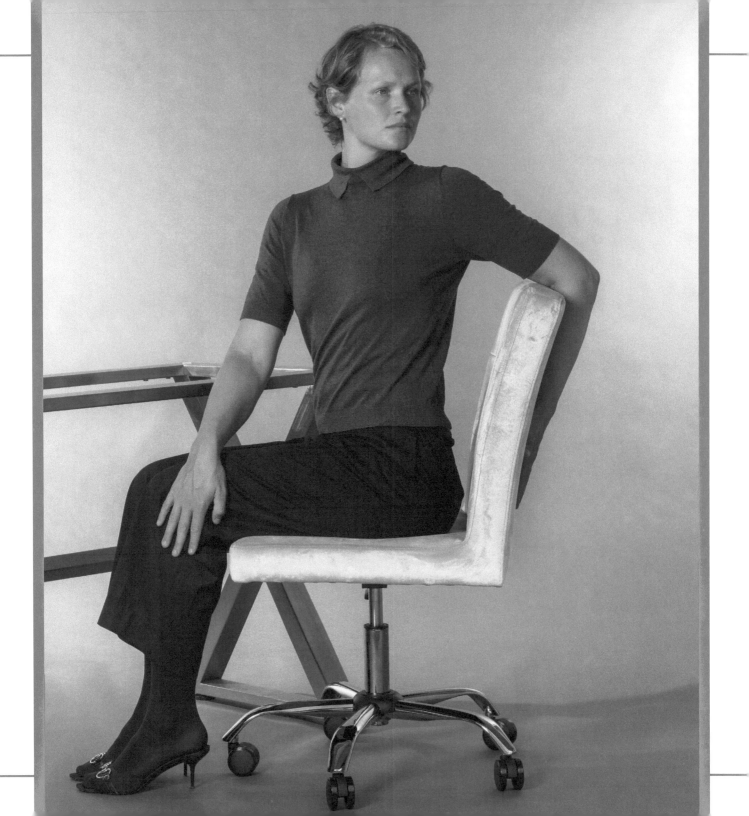

CHAPTER 4:

THE EXERCISES: DAILY
WORKDAY SEQUENCE[8]

Postural improvement and maintenance are best done if practiced in short segments, several times a day. You must make working on your posture a habit.

The following posture yoga sequence is designed to counteract the effects of forward slumping and can be performed once through in 10 to 15 minutes in your work or home office during your workday. It is intended to supplement (not replace) your gym or other outside-office exercise routine. By performing these exercises one or more times a day during your workday, you will not only continue to improve your posture but also increase your awareness of your postural alignment, which will help you to self-correct any future misalignment.

Before starting any of the seated exercises, be sure that you are sitting properly in your chair. Proper sitting alignment includes sitting up straight, resting both feet flat on the floor while keeping your knees level with your hips and sitting back in your chair so that your lower back is supported by the back of the chair.

---

8 Always consult your physician before beginning any exercise program. This general information is not intended to diagnose any medical condition or to replace your healthcare professional. If you experience any pain or difficulty with these exercises, stop and consult your healthcare provider.

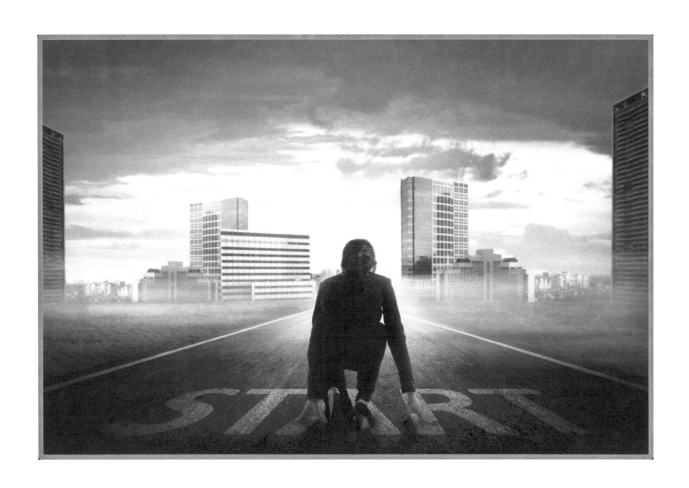

Daily Workday Posture Yoga Sequence – 10 exercises (10-15 minutes to perform all 10)

Daily Exercise #1 – Interlace Fingers Behind Back

Purpose – Opens the chest, releases tension in the shoulders

Exercise Cues

- Sit at the front of your chair.

- Interlace your fingers behind your back.

- Inhale as you sit tall and lengthen your torso.

- Exhale as you squeeze your shoulder blades together and slightly tuck your tailbone under while drawing in your abdomen.

- Repeat 5 times.

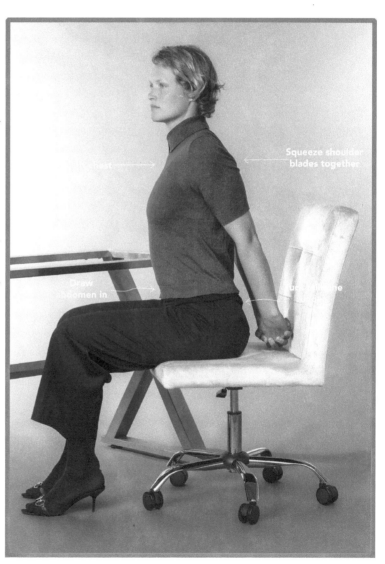

Daily Exercise #2 – Classic Yoga Chair

Purpose – Opens the chest and shoulders, strengthens the back, tones the thighs

Exercise Cues

- Stand with feet hip-width apart in front of your chair.

- Reach both hands up above you, palms facing each other, as if you were trying to touch the ceiling, and drop your shoulders.

- Keeping the straight line from the base of your tailbone up to the tips of your fingers, slowly reach your glutes back, as if you were going to sit into your chair (but do not) and drop your tailbone.

- Hold this position for 5 breaths, inhaling as you arch your chest slightly forward, and exhaling as you squeeze your shoulder blades together while grounding your weight in your heels.

- After 5 breaths, stand up and repeat this exercise 2 more times.

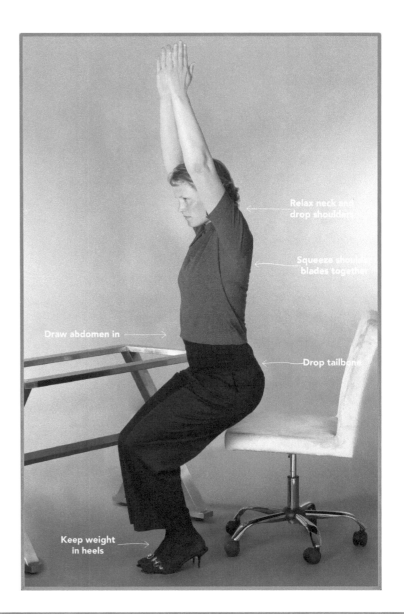

Relax neck and drop shoulders

Squeeze shoulder blades together

Draw abdomen in

Drop tailbone

Keep weight in heels

Daily Exercise #3 – Shoulder Blade Squeeze

Purpose – Opens the chest and strengthens the upper and mid back

Exercise Cues

- Sit with both feet planted firmly on the floor.

- Extend your arms out at your sides, as if you were trying to touch the walls on either side of you, palms facing down.

- Slightly bend your elbows.

- Lean your upper body forward approximately 45 degrees.

- Holding this position, inhale and lengthen your spine, then exhale and squeeze your shoulder blades together, as if you were squeezing a pencil between them.

- Hold the squeeze for 3 seconds.

- Perform 10 squeezes, holding each for 3 seconds.

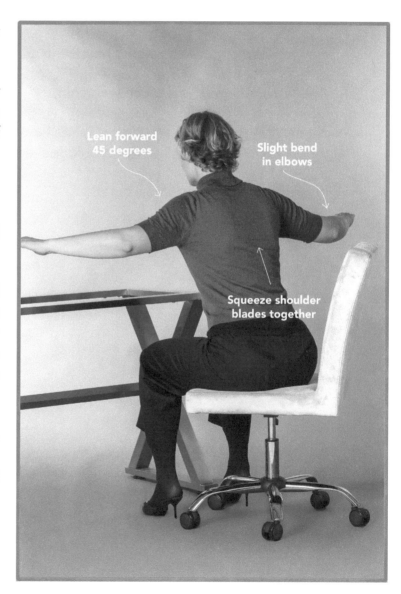

Lean forward 45 degrees

Slight bend in elbows

Squeeze shoulder blades together

Daily Exercise #4 – Chin Tucks

Purpose – Helps improve your neck's strength and flexibility. Important exercise for keeping your head aligned with your spine. Mitigates forward-head jut.

Exercise Cues

- Sit facing forward and look straight ahead with your ears directly over your shoulders.

- Take one of your fingers and touch your chin.

- Without moving your finger, separate your chin away from your finger by pulling your chin straight back toward your neck. You should feel a stretch at the back of the neck.

- Hold this stretch for 5 slow, deep breaths.

- Perform this exercise 3 times.

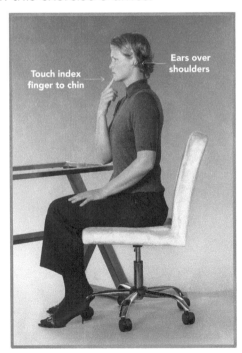
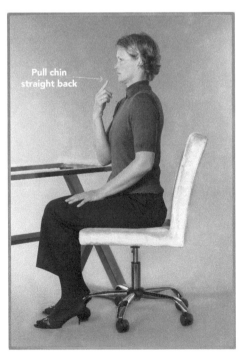

Purpose – Opens the front body, including chest and ribs. Eases tension in the shoulders. Tones the back and abdomen

Exercise Cues

- Straighten your arms at your sides and turn your palms up to face the ceiling.

- Inhale as you raise your arms above your head and bring your palms to touch.

- Reach your arms higher toward the ceiling as you push your shoulders back, keeping your neck straight.

- Exhale your arms down as you draw your abdomen in and tuck your tailbone under slightly.

- Repeat 10 times.

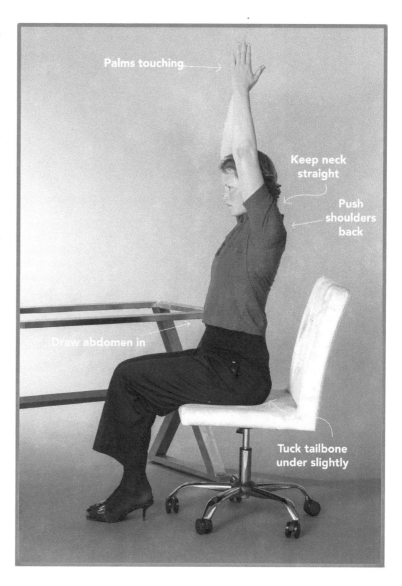

Palms touching

Keep neck straight

Push shoulders back

Draw abdomen in

Tuck tailbone under slightly

Daily Exercise #6 – Side Stretch with Raised Arms

Purpose – Stretches the side body, including the muscles between your ribs. Improves spinal flexibility.

Exercise Cues

- Inhale as you reach your arms straight above your head.

- Grab your left wrist with your right hand.

- Exhale as you pull your left arm toward your right side, keeping your left arm straight as you lean to your right.

- You should feel a stretch in your left side-body.

- Take 5 breaths holding the stretch, lengthening your right side-body on each inhale, and deepening your lean to the right on each exhale.

- Switch arms and repeat on the other side.

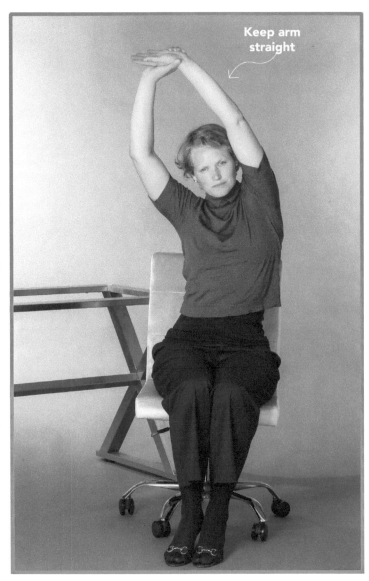

Keep arm straight

Daily Exercise #7 – Seated Twist

Purpose – Increases flexibility in the spine and back, stretches shoulders and chest

Exercise Cues

- Sit back in your chair, facing forward with both feet flat on the floor.

- Twist to the right and place your left palm on the outside of your right thigh and your right hand on the back of your chair.

- Inhale and lengthen your torso.

- Exhale and push your left hand into your right thigh and revolve your upper torso toward the right.

- Hold for three breaths, lengthening your spine on the inhale, and revolving more deeply to your right on the exhale.

- Repeat on the left side.

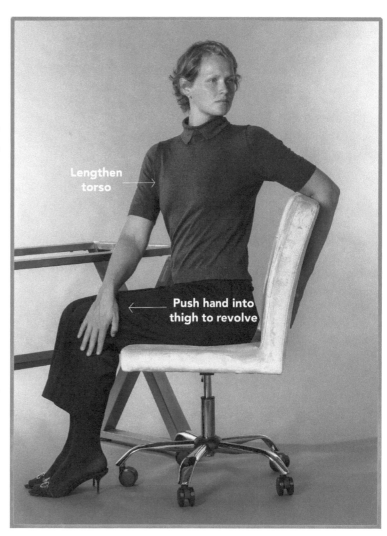

Daily Exercise #8 – Seated Lunge

Purpose – Tight hip flexors can cause lower back pain. This exercise improves flexibility in the hip flexors and quads

Exercise Cues

- Sit upright with your left thigh and glute muscle fully on the chair seat, keeping your left foot flat and your left knee directly above your left foot.

- Slide your right leg off the chair and extend it straight behind you as far as you comfortably can, keeping the ball of your right foot on the floor.

- Lean back.

- Hold this position for 5 breaths, contracting your glutes on each inhale, and pulling your abdomen in on each exhale.

- You should feel your right hip flexor and quad stretch.

- Repeat on the other leg.

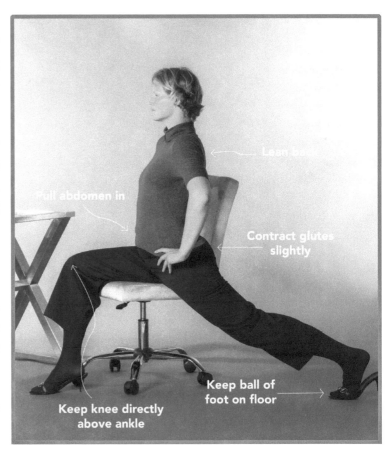

Lean back

Pull abdomen in

Contract glutes slightly

Keep knee directly above ankle

Keep ball of foot on floor

Daily Exercise #9 – Hamstring Stretch

Purpose – Stretches hamstrings

Exercise Cues

- Place your left foot flat on the floor and bend your left knee at a right angle to the chair, keeping your left knee directly over your left foot.

- Stretch your right leg out in front of you, keeping your right heel on the floor.

- Place your hands on your hips and inhale as you lengthen your spine.

- Keeping your right leg straight, exhale as you gently bend at the hips toward your right foot. For increased stretch, flex your right foot as you bend toward your right foot.

- You should feel this stretch in your hamstrings, behind your thigh and knee.

- Hold for 5 breaths, lengthening your spine on each inhale and deepening the stretch on each exhale.

- Repeat on the other leg.

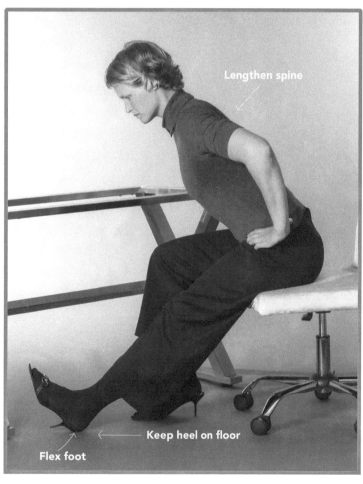

Daily Exercise #10 – Chest Stretch at Wall or in Doorframe

Purpose – Stretches the pectoralis muscles of the chest

Exercise Cues

- Stand facing the wall or doorframe and place your right forearm flat against the wall or a doorframe, with your elbow at 90 degrees.

- Keeping your arm here, shift your weight to your left and rotate your body as far as you can to your left, pivoting away from the wall/doorframe.

- Hold for 10 breaths, deepening the stretch as you breathe into the hold.

- Repeat on the other side.

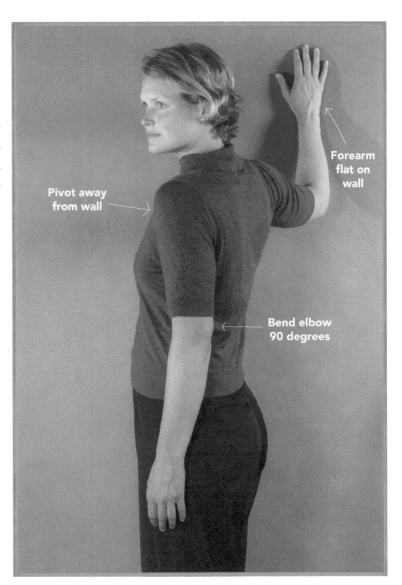

Pivot away from wall

Forearm flat on wall

Bend elbow 90 degrees

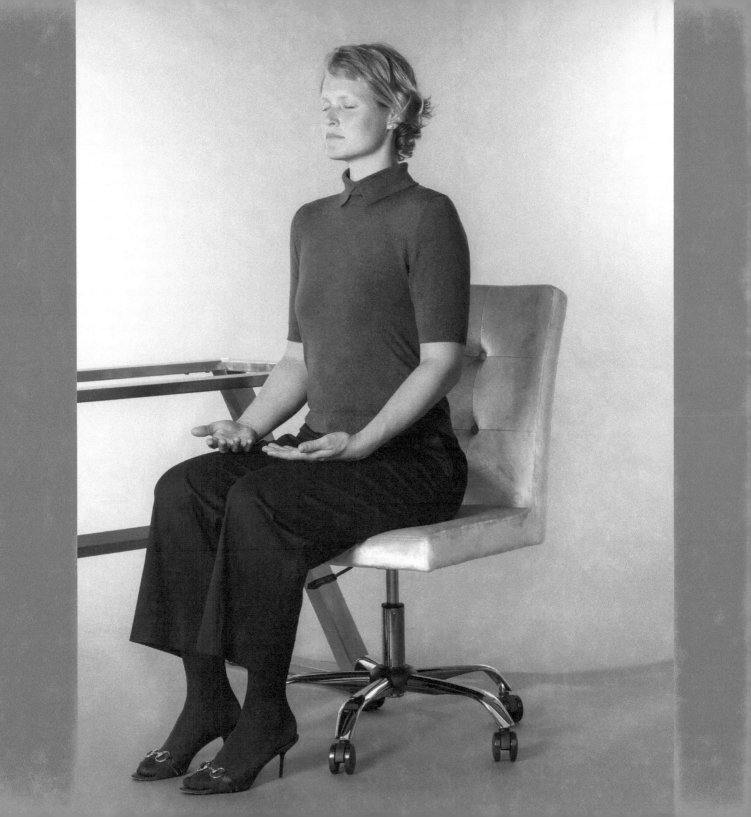

CHAPTER 5:
BONUS EXERCISES

The previous set of 10 exercises should be performed every day. If you have additional time, below are some bonus exercises to supplement the 10 daily exercises.

Bonus #1 - Chairback Grabs

Purpose – Opens the chest, releases tension in the shoulders

Exercise Cues

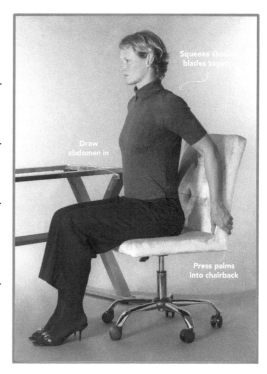

- Look straight ahead.

- Hook the palms of your hands on the back of your chair's seat.

- Walk your hands close to each other so that your elbows are directly behind you and above your wrists.

- Inhale as you lengthen your sternum and press your palms into the back of the chair's seat.

- Exhale as you draw your shoulder blades together, bring your elbows closer together, and draw your abdomen in.

- Repeat 10 times.

Bonus #2 - Seated Reverse Prayer

Purpose – Opens up the chest and shoulders, stretches wrists

Exercise Cues

Option 1 (Basic):

- Make two fists and bring your fists behind your back, pressing them as close together as you can.

- Holding this position, inhale as you expand across your chest and roll your shoulders back.

- Exhale as you press your elbows back and your fists together, while drawing your abdomen in.

- Perform this exercise for 5 breaths.

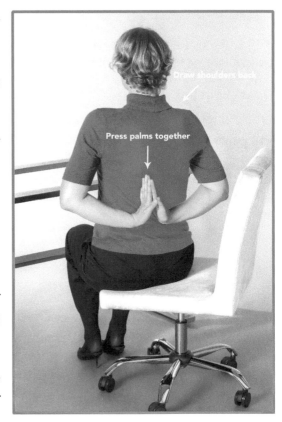

Option 2 (Advanced):

- Bring your arms behind your back and join your palms together, keeping your fingers pointing downward.

- Next, rotate your fingertips inward toward the spine until your fingertips point upward with your palms joined together.

- Holding this position, inhale as you expand across your chest and roll your shoulders back.

- Exhale as your press your palms together and draw your abdomen in.

- Hold this position for 5 breaths.

Bonus #3 - Arm Raise with Elbow Grab

Purpose – Opens chest and shoulders

Exercise Cues

- Inhale as you raise both your arms above your head.

- Exhale and grab each elbow with the opposite hand, framing your face with your arms.

- Inhale as you arch your chest forward and open, bringing your shoulders back.

- Exhale as you return to sitting up straight, lengthening your spine, and drawing your abdomen in. Repeat 10 times.

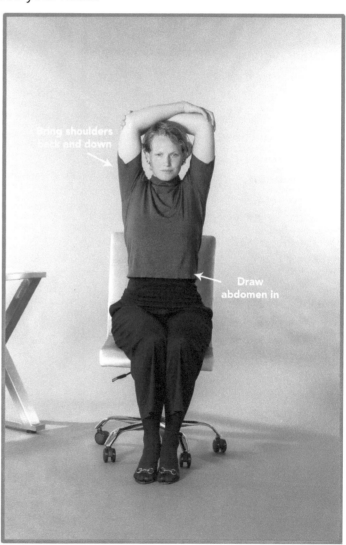

Bring shoulders back and down

Draw abdomen in

Bonus #4 - Triceps Stretch

Purpose – Opens the shoulders and chest, stretches triceps

Exercise Cues

- Raise your right arm above your head.

- Bend your right arm at the elbow, bringing the right palm of your hand to touch your upper back.

- Inhale and use your left hand to pull your right elbow closer to your head.

- Exhale as you walk your right hand's fingertips lower down your back.

- Press your head back slightly into your upper arm.

- Take 5 deep breaths here.

- Repeat on the left arm.

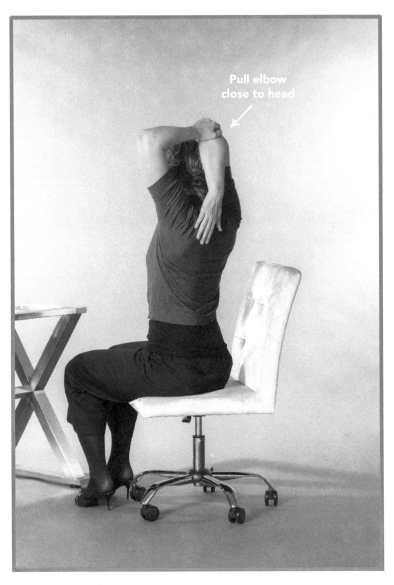

Pull elbow close to head

Purpose – Releases tension in the shoulders and upper back

Exercise Cues

- Bring your right arm across your chest, keeping it straight.

- Press your left hand into your right arm toward your chest.

- Inhale and lengthen your sternum.

- Exhale and press your left hand into your right arm.

- Take 5 breaths here, lengthening your sternum on each inhale and pressing into your right arm on each exhale.

- Repeat exercise on the left arm.

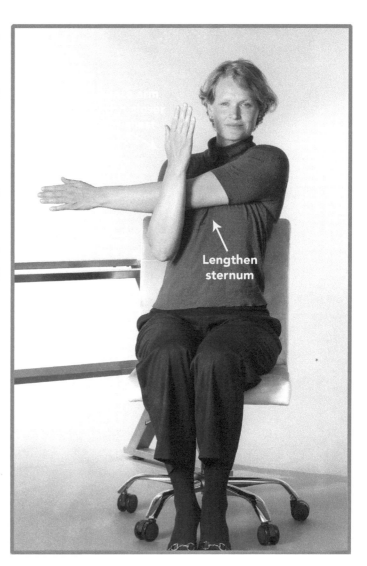

Lengthen sternum

Purpose – Stretches the back of the neck and shoulders

Exercise Cues

- Cross your arms so that your right elbow is on top of your left elbow.

- Place your hands on your shoulder blades (or as close as you can get).

- Inhale and raise your elbows.

- Exhale and lower your elbows.

- Repeat 5 times.

- Switch arm positions and repeat with left elbow on top of the right elbow.

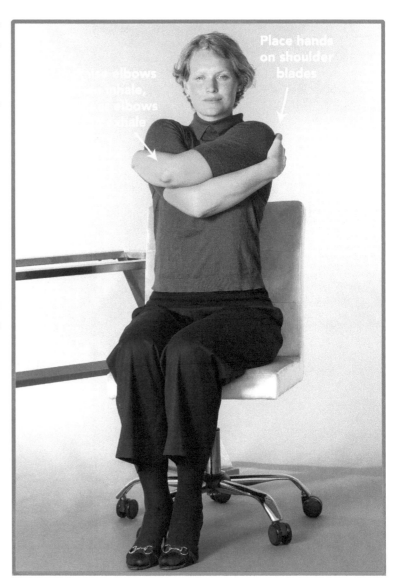

Purpose – Loosens up and releases tension in the shoulders

Exercise Cues

- Inhale as you move your shoulders up and back, broadening across your chest as you draw your shoulder blades together.

- Exhale as you move your shoulders down and forward, broadening across your upper back while contracting your chest.

- Repeat for 10 breaths.

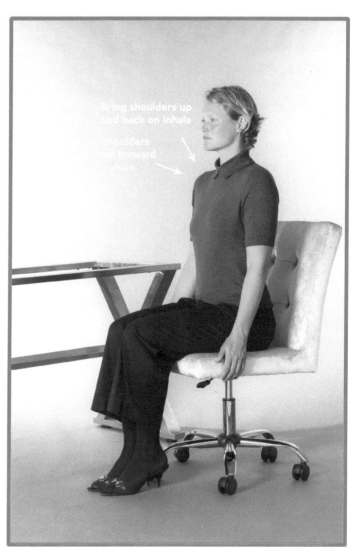

Bonus #8 - Neck Rotation

Purpose – Stretches the sides of the neck

Exercise Cues

Do this exercise slowly. If this movement causes pain at any time, stop immediately.

- Look straight ahead.

- Keeping your shoulders square in front of you, inhale and slowly turn your head to face the right.

- Exhale and slowly turn your head to face the left. Return to face forward.

- Repeat for 5 breaths.

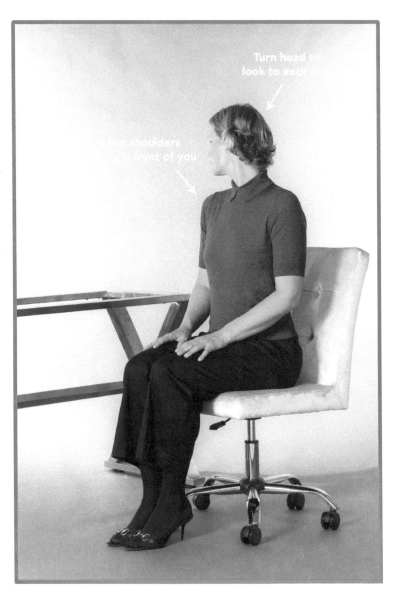

Turn head to look to each side

Keep shoulders square in front of you

Bonus #9 - Neck Side Stretch

Purpose – Stretches the sides of the neck

Exercise Cues

Do this exercise slowly. If this movement causes pain at any time, stop immediately.

- Bend your right arm at a right angle at your side with right palm facing up, keeping your elbow close to your torso.

- Place your left hand on the top of your head and slowly tilt your left ear toward your left shoulder.

- Slowly apply gentle pressure with your left hand to increase the stretch.

- Hold for 5 breaths.

- Repeat on the other side.

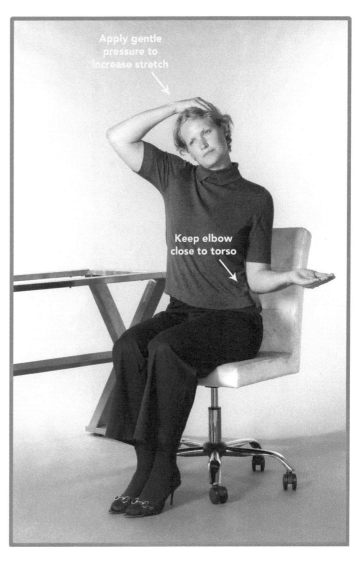

Apply gentle pressure to increase stretch

Keep elbow close to torso

Bonus #10 - Seated Leg Raises

Purpose – Strengthens the core, including lower abs. Improves flexibility of the abdomen and hips.

Exercise Cues

- Sit so that your low back touches the back of the chair and press your palms down on your chair on either side of your legs.

- Inhale and stretch your legs out in front of you, and pull your abdomen in.

- Keeping your abdomen in and your core braced in this position, exhale as you lift both of your straight legs as high as comfortable.

- Inhale as you lower your legs, keeping your abdomen braced pulling in.

- Repeat raising both legs and lowering them slowly for 10 breaths.

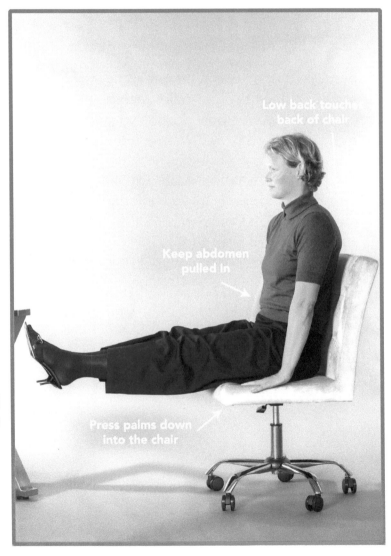

Low back touches back of chair

Keep abdomen pulled in

Press palms down into the chair

Purpose – Reduces mental tension and promotes self-awareness

Exercise Cues

- Sit back in your chair so that your low back is touching the back of the chair.

- Place your palms face up on your thighs.

- Look straight ahead and close your eyes.

- Picture in your mind a relaxing, peaceful scene, such as a still lake.

- Focus on this image as you listen to your breath for 10 breaths.

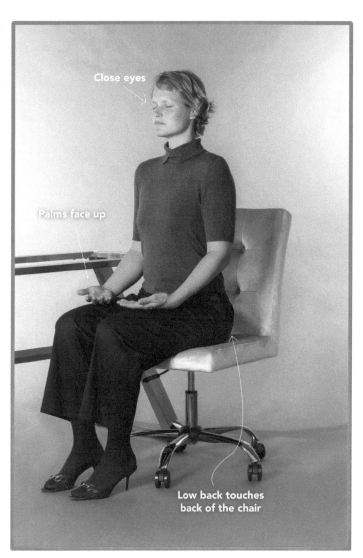

Close eyes

Palms face up

Low back touches
back of the chair

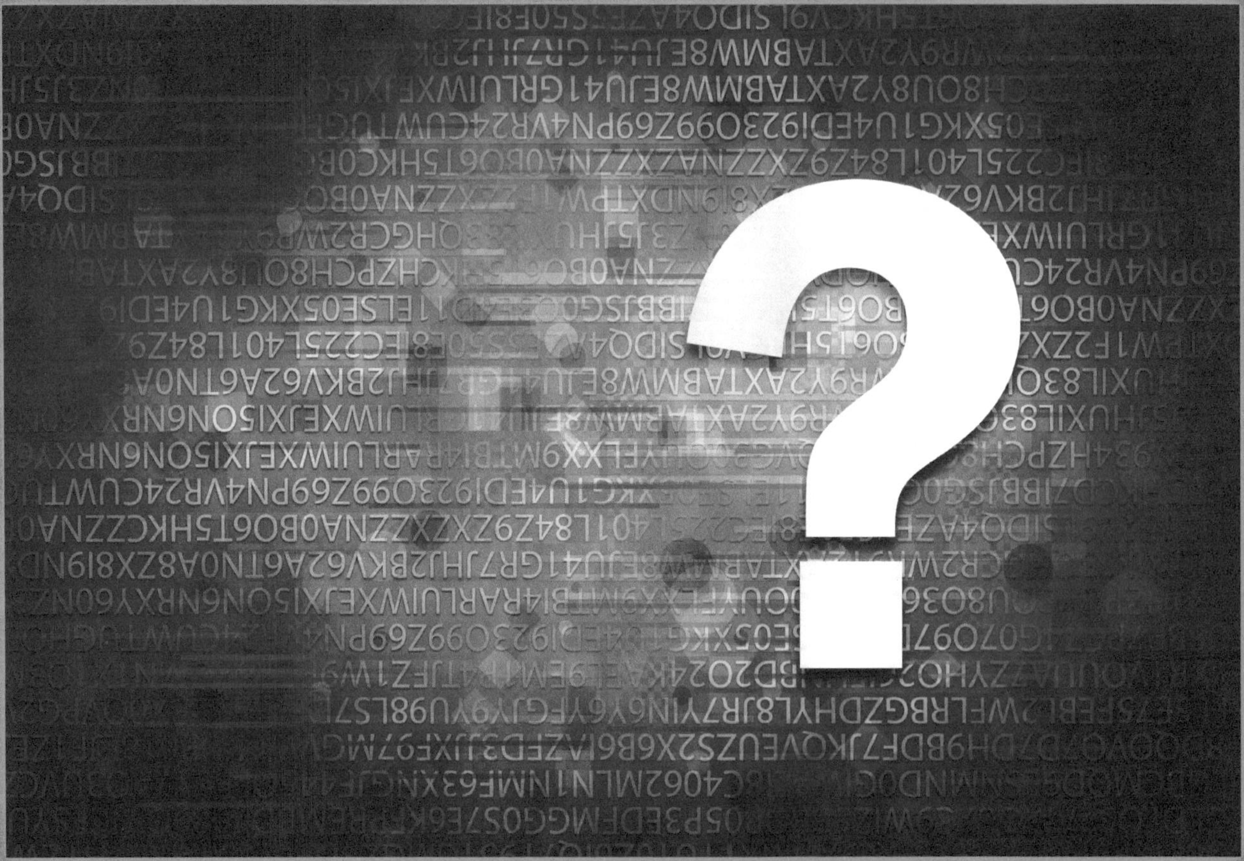

CHAPTER 6:
COMMON QUESTIONS ABOUT THE EXERCISES (WITH ANSWERS)

The following are some common questions and answers about the recommended exercises.

1. **Do I really have to do the exercises every day?**
   Answer: Yes, if you would like to achieve results of acquiring good posture and then maintaining it, we recommend that you do the 10 daily workday exercises every day. A daily cadence will retrain and reinforce your muscles' proper alignment.

2. **Once I get good at the exercises, do I have to keep doing them?**
   Answer: Yes, the key to success in maintaining good posture is flexibility and strength, and we all have to continue to work at these.

3. **Ideally, how many times a day should I do these exercises?**
   Answer: Ideally, you should do the set of 10 daily workday exercises at least twice a day.

4. **I go to the gym every day. Do I still have to do these exercises?**
   Answer: Yes. We recommend that these exercises supplement any fitness routine you might have.

5. **What happens if I miss a day or don't have time to do all 10 of the daily exercises?**
   Answer: Try to do whatever you have time for and resume the full program whenever you can.

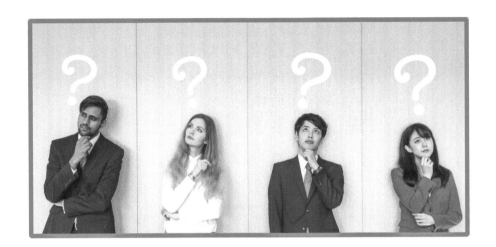

6. **Do I have to do the breathing that is cued as part of the exercises?**
Answer: We recommend that you take deep, slow breaths and do the breathing as cued in the exercises. Breathing causes the movement of energy and helps the body relax. You will feel much more relaxed and invigorated if you do and pay attention to the breathing as cued in the exercises.

7. **What does it mean when it says that I am supposed to hold an exercise for a certain number of breaths?**
Answer: One breath is a complete cycle of an inhale followed by an exhale. The breath in each exercise should be deep and even. Try to make each inhale and exhale 3 or 4 seconds each.

8. **When should I do the bonus exercises?**
Answer: Do the bonus exercises after you have done all 10 of the daily workday exercises if you have time to do more.

9. **Can I do these if I've had back surgery?**
Answer: Before starting any new exercise program, consult your doctor. Go slowly and do the exercises gently. If a seated twist or any other exercise causes discomfort, slow down and do not be as vigorous. If you experience any pain or difficulty with these exercises, stop and consult your healthcare provider.

APPENDIX:

REFERENCE SHEETS TO POST AT YOUR DESK

The following are cheat-sheet references (both picture and list formats) that you can post at your desk to remind you of the summary cues for the 10 essential exercises (and bonus exercises if you have time).

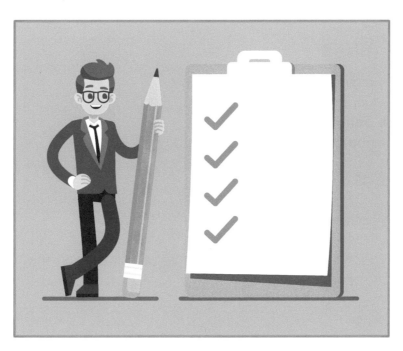

THE PROFESSIONAL POSTURE PROGRAM:
DAILY SEQUENCE -- REFERENCE SHEET

1. **Interlace Fingers Behind Back**
   - *Inhale* as you lift your chest.

   - *Exhale* as you squeeze your shoulder blades together, slightly tuck your tailbone under and draw abdomen in.

   - Repeat for 5 breaths.

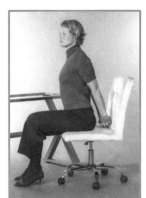

2. **Classic Yoga Chair**
   - Stand and raise arms above you, reach glutes back, and drop your tailbone.

   - Hold the position for 5 breaths. On each *inhale*, arch your chest forward. On each *exhale*, squeeze your shoulder blades together.

   - Stand after 5 breaths.

   - Do 3 times, holding for 5 breaths each time.

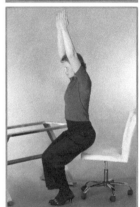

3. **Shoulder Blade Squeeze**
   - Extend arms out at sides, slightly bend elbows.

   - Lean forward 45 degrees.

   - *Inhale* and lengthen your spine.

   - *Exhale* and squeeze your shoulder blades together, holding the squeeze for 3 seconds.

   - Perform 10 times.

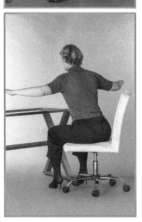

4. **Chin Tucks**
   - *Inhale* as you sit up straight in a chair with ears over shoulders and touch your index finger to your chin.
   - Without moving your finger, *exhale* and pull your chin straight back toward the neck and hold for 5 breaths.
   - Repeat exercise 3 times.

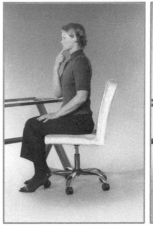 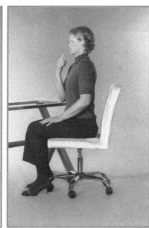

5. **Arm Raise**
   - *Inhale* as you raise your arms above you, palms together, reaching arms toward the ceiling as you push your shoulders back. Keep neck straight.
   - *Exhale* as you lower your arms, draw your abdomen in and tuck your tailbone under slightly.
   - Repeat 10 times.

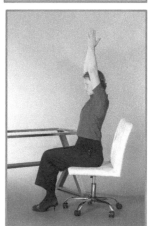

6. **Side Stretch with Raised Arms**
   - Grab your left wrist with your right hand and pull your left arm toward your right side, keeping your left arm straight as you lean right.
   - Hold this position for 5 breaths. On each *inhale*, lengthen your side body. On each *exhale*, deepen your lean.
   - Repeat on the other side.

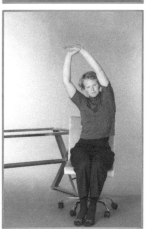

7. Seated Twist

- Place your left palm on your right thigh and your right hand on the back of your chair.

- *Inhale* and lengthen your torso.

- *Exhale* and twist to the right.

- Hold for 3 breaths, lengthening your torso on each inhale and deepening the twist on each exhale.

- Repeat on the other side.

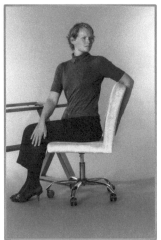

8. Seated Lunge

- Sit with your left thigh and glute muscle on the chair, keeping your left knee directly above your left foot.

- Slide your right leg off the chair and extend it directly behind you, keeping the ball of your right foot on the floor. Lean back.

- *Inhale* as you contract your glutes, and *exhale* as you pull your abdomen in and lean back slightly more. Hold for 5 breaths.

- Repeat on the other leg.

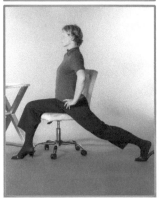

9. Hamstring Stretch

- Place your left foot on the floor, with your left knee directly over your left foot. Stretch your right leg out in front of you.

- *Inhale* and lengthen your spine. *Exhale* and bend forward at the hips, drawing your abdomen in and squeezing the shoulder blades together.

- Hold for 5 breaths. Repeat on the other leg.

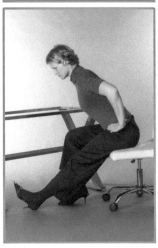

10. **Chest Stretch at Wall or in Doorframe**

- Place your right forearm flat against the wall, with your elbow at 90 degrees.

- *Inhale* and lengthen your spine. *Exhale* and rotate your body as far as you can to the left, pivoting away from the wall.

- Hold for 10 breaths. Deepen your stretch as you breathe.

- Repeat on the other side.

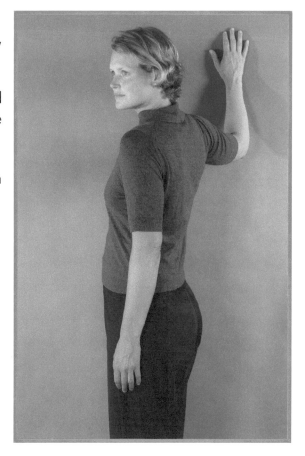

Bonus Exercises (Time Permitting) – Reference Sheet

Bonus - #1. Chairback Grabs

- Hook the palms of your hands on the back of the chair's seat.
- Walk your hands close to each other so that your elbows are directly behind you and above your wrists.
- *Inhale* and lengthen your sternum as you press your palms into the chair seat.
- *Exhale* as you draw your shoulder blades together.
- Perform for 10 breaths.

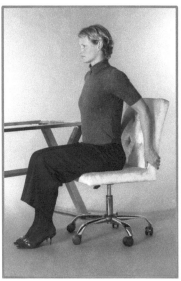

Bonus #2. Seated Reverse Prayer

Option 1 - Basic

- Make two fists and bring your fists behind your back, pressing them as close together as you can.
- *Inhale* as you expand across your chest.
- *Exhale* and press your elbows back and draw your abdomen in.
- Perform for 5 breaths.

Option 2 - Advanced

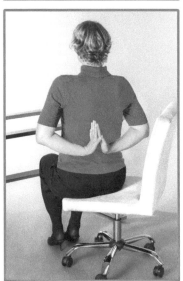

- Bring your arms behind your back and join your palms together, pointing your fingers downward.
- Rotate your fingertips inward toward the spine until your fingertips point upward with your palms joined together.
- *Inhale* as you expand across your chest.
- *Exhale* as your press your palms together and draw your abdomen in.
- Perform for 5 breaths.

Bonus #3. Arm Raise with Elbow Grab

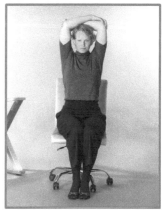

- *Inhale* and raise both arms above your head.
- *Exhale* and grab each elbow with the opposite hand, framing your face with your arms.
- *Inhale* and arch your chest forward and open, bringing your shoulders back.
- *Exhale* as you return to sitting up straight, lengthening your spine, and drawing your navel in.
- Repeat 10 times.

Bonus #4. Triceps Stretch

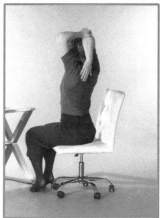

- Raise your right arm above your head and bend it at the elbow, bringing the palm of your hand to touch your upper back.
- *Inhale* and use your left hand to pull your right elbow closer to your head.
- *Exhale* as you walk your right hand's fingertips lower down your back. Press your head back slightly into your upper arm.
- Take 5 deep breaths here.
- Repeat on the left arm.

Bonus #5. Arm Cross Stretch

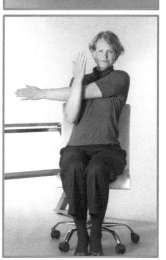

- Bring your right arm across your chest, keeping it straight.
- Press your left hand into your right arm toward your chest.
- *Inhale* and lengthen your sternum.
- *Exhale* and press your left hand into your right arm.
- Take 5 breaths here, lengthening your sternum on each inhale, pressing into your right arm on each exhale.
- Switch arms and repeat.

Bonus #6. Self Embrace

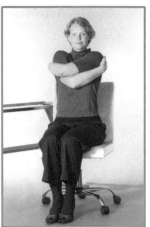

- Cross your arms so your right elbow is on top of your left elbow.

- Place your hands on your shoulder blades (or as close as you can).

- *Inhale* and raise your elbows.

- *Exhale* and lower your elbows. Perform 5 times.

- Change arms and repeat on the other side with left elbow on top.

Bonus #7. Shoulder Rolls

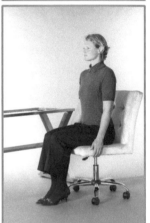

- *Inhale* as you move your shoulders up and back, broadening across your chest as you draw your shoulder blades together.

- *Exhale* as you move your shoulders down and forward, broadening across your upper back while contracting your chest.

- Repeat for 10 breaths.

Bonus #8. Neck Rotation

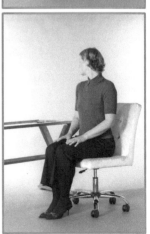

Do this exercise slowly. If this movement causes pain at any time, stop immediately.

- Look straight ahead. Keep your shoulders square in front of you.

- Inhale and slowly turn your head to the right.

- *Exhale* and slowly turn your head to the left.

- Return to face forward. Repeat for 5 breaths.

Bonus #9. Neck Side Stretch

Do this exercise slowly. If this movement causes pain at any time, stop immediately.

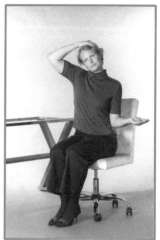

- Bend your right arm at a right angle at your side with right palm facing up, keeping your elbow close to your torso.
- Place your left hand on the top of your head and slowly tilt your left ear toward your left shoulder.
- Slowly apply gentle pressure with your left hand to increase the stretch.
- Hold for 5 breaths. Repeat on the other side.

Bonus #10. Seated Leg Raise

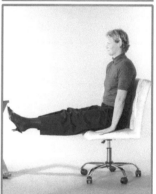

- Sit so that your low back touches the back of the chair.
- Press your palms down on either side of your legs.
- *Inhale* and stretch your legs out in front of you, as you pull your abdomen in.
- Keeping your abdomen in and your core braced in this position, *exhale* and lift both of your legs as high as you comfortably can.
- *Inhale* as you lower your legs, keeping your abdomen braced, pulling in.
- Repeat raising both legs and lowering them slowly for 10 breaths.

Bonus #11. Seated Meditation

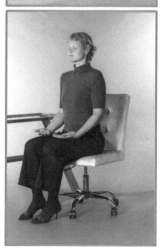

- Sit so that your low back is touching the back of the chair.
- Place your palms face up on your thighs.
- Look straight ahead and close your eyes.
- Picture in your mind a relaxing, peaceful scene, such as a still lake.
- Focus only on this image as you listen to your breath for 10 slow, deep breaths.

Professional Posture Program: Daily Workday Exercise List

*Unless otherwise noted, perform each exercise while seated in your chair.

	Exercise	Cues	# of Reps
1.	**Interlace Fingers Behind Back**	• Interlace your fingers behind your back. • *Inhale* as you lift your chest. • *Exhale* as you squeeze your shoulder blades together, slightly tuck your tailbone under and draw abdomen in.	Perform for 5 breaths.
2.	**Classic Yoga Chair***	• Stand and raise arms above you, reach glutes back. • *Inhale* as you arch your chest forward. • *Exhale* as you squeeze your shoulder blades together.	Perform 3 times, holding each for 5 breaths.
3.	**Shoulder Blade Squeeze**	• Extend arms out at sides, slightly bend elbows, and lean forward 45 degrees. • *Inhale* and lengthen your spine. • *Exhale* and squeeze your shoulder blades together.	Perform 10 times, holding each squeeze for 3 seconds.
4.	**Chin Tucks**	• *Inhale* as you sit up straight with ears over shoulders and touch your index finger to your chin. • *Exhale* and pull your chin away from your finger and straight back toward the back of the neck and hold the stretch.	Perform 3 times, holding each stretch for 5 breaths.

5.	Arm Raise	• *Inhale* as you raise your arms above you, palms together, reaching arms toward the ceiling as you push your shoulders back. Keep neck straight. • *Exhale* as you lower your arms, draw your abdomen in and tuck your tailbone under slightly.	Perform 10 times.
6. Right Side	Side Stretch with Raised Arms – Right Side Stretch	• Grab your **left** wrist with your **right** hand and pull your left arm toward your **right** side, keeping your **left** arm straight as you lean **right**. • *Inhale* as you lengthen your **left** side-body. • *Exhale* as you deepen your lean to the **right**.	Hold for 5 breaths.
6. Left Side	Side Stretch with Raised Arms – Left Side Stretch	• Grab your **right** wrist with your **left** hand and pull your **right** arm toward your **left** side, keeping your **right** arm straight as you lean **left**. • *Inhale* as you lengthen your **right** side-body. • *Exhale* as you deepen your lean to the **left**.	Hold for 5 breaths.
7. Right Side	Seated Twist– Right Side Stretch	• Place the **left** palm on the **right** thigh and **right** hand on the back of your chair. • *Inhale* and lengthen your torso. • *Exhale* and twist to the **right**.	Hold for 3 breaths.

7. **Left** **Side**	**Seated** **Twist– Left** **Side Stretch**	• Place the **right** palm on the **left** thigh and **left** hand on the back of your chair. • *Inhale* and lengthen your torso. • *Exhale* and twist to the **left**.	Hold for 3 breaths.
8. **Right** **Side**	**Seated** **Lunge–** **Right Side** **Stretch**	• Sit with your **left** thigh and glute muscle on the chair, keeping your **left** knee directly above your **left** foot. • Slide your **right** leg off the chair and extend it behind you, keeping the ball of your **right** foot on the floor. Lean back. • *Inhale* as your contract your glutes. • *Exhale* as you pull your abdomen in and lean back slightly more.	Hold for 5 breaths.
8. **Left** **Side**	**Seated** **Lunge– Left** **Side Stretch**	• Sit with your **right** thigh and glute muscle on the chair, keeping your **right** knee directly above your **right** foot. • Slide your **left** leg off the chair and extend it behind you, keeping the ball of your **left** foot on the floor. Lean back. • *Inhale* as your contract your glutes. • *Exhale* as you pull your abdomen in and lean back slightly more.	Hold for 5 breaths.

9. Right Side	**Hamstring Stretch– Right Side Stretch**	• Place your **left** foot on the floor, with your **left** knee directly over your **left** foot. • Stretch your **right** leg out in front of you. • *Inhale* and lengthen your spine. • *Exhale* as you bend forward at the hips, drawing the abdomen in and squeezing shoulder blades together.	Hold for 5 breaths.
9. Left Side	**Hamstring Stretch– Left Side Stretch**	• Place your **right** foot on the floor, with your **right** knee directly over your **right** foot. • Stretch your **left** leg out in front of you. • *Inhale* and lengthen your spine. • *Exhale* as you bend forward at the hips, drawing the abdomen in and squeezing shoulder blades together.	Hold for 5 breaths.
10. Right Side	**Chest Stretch at Wall or Doorframe– Right Side Stretch***	• Standing at the wall, place your **right** forearm flat against the wall, with your elbow at 90 degrees. • *Inhale* and lengthen your spine. • *Exhale* and rotate your body as far as you can to the **left**, pivoting away from the wall.	Hold for 10 breaths.

10. Left Side	Chest Stretch at Wall or Doorframe– Left Side Stretch*	• Standing at the wall, place your **left** forearm flat against the wall, with your elbow at 90 degrees. • *Inhale* and lengthen your spine. • *Exhale* and rotate your body as far as you can to the **right**, pivoting away from the wall.	Hold for 10 breaths.

Bonus Exercises
(if time permits)

Perform each bonus exercise while seated in your chair.

	Exercise	Cues	# of Reps
Bonus #1	**Chairback Grabs**	• Hook the palms of your hands on the back of the chair's seat. • Walk your hands close to each other so that your elbows are directly behind you and above your wrists. • *Inhale* and lengthen your sternum as you press your palms into the chair seat. • *Exhale* as you draw your shoulder blades together.	Perform for 10 breaths.
Bonus #2	**Seated Reverse Prayer**	• *Option 1 - Basic:* Make two fists and bring your fists behind your back, pressing them as close together as you can. • *Option 2 – Advanced:* Bring your arms behind your back and join your palms together, pointing your fingers downward. Rotate your fingertips inward toward the spine until your fingertips point upward with your palms joined together. • *Inhale* as you expand across your chest. • *Exhale* as your press your palms together and draw your abdomen in.	Perform for 5 breaths.

Bonus #3	**Arm Raise with Elbow Grab**	• Raise both arms above your head. Grab each elbow with the opposite hand, framing your face with your arms. • *Inhale* and arch your chest forward and open, bringing your shoulders back. • *Exhale* as you return to sitting up straight, lengthening your spine, and drawing your navel in.	Perform for 10 breaths.
Bonus #4 Right Side	**Triceps Stretch – Right Arm**	• Raise your **right** arm above your head and bend it at the elbow, bringing the palm of your hand to touch your upper back. • *Inhale* and use your **left** hand to pull your right elbow closer to your head. • *Exhale* as you walk your **right** hand's fingertips lower down your back. Press your head back slightly into your upper arm.	Hold for 5 breaths.
Bonus #4 Left Side	**Triceps Stretch – Left Arm**	• Raise your **left** arm above your head and bend it at the elbow, bringing the palm of your hand to touch your upper back. • *Inhale* and use your **right** hand to pull your right elbow closer to your head. • *Exhale* as you walk your **left** hand's fingertips lower down your back. Press your head back slightly into your upper arm.	Hold for 5 breaths.

Bonus #5 Right Side	**Arm Cross Stretch – Right Arm**	• Bring your **right** arm across your chest, keeping it straight. • Press your **left** hand into your **right** arm toward your chest. • *Inhale* and lengthen your sternum. • *Exhale* and press your **left** hand into your **right** arm.	Hold for 5 breaths.
Bonus #5 Left Side	**Arm Cross Stretch – Left Arm**	• Bring your **left** arm across your chest, keeping it straight. • Press your **right** hand into your **left** arm toward your chest. • *Inhale* and lengthen your sternum. • *Exhale* and press your **right** hand into your **left** arm.	Hold for 5 breaths.
Bonus #6 Right Arm on Top	**Self Embrace – Right Arm on Top**	• Cross your arms so your **right** elbow is on top of your **left** elbow. • Place your hands on your shoulder blades (or as close as you can). • *Inhale* and raise your elbows. • *Exhale* and lower your elbows.	Perform for 5 breaths.

Bonus #6 Left Arm on Top	**Self Embrace – Left Arm on Top**	• Cross your arms so your **left** elbow is on top of your **right** elbow. • Place your hands on your shoulder blades (or as close as you can). • *Inhale* and raise your elbows. • *Exhale* and lower your elbows.	Perform for 5 breaths.
Bonus #7	**Shoulder Rolls**	• *Inhale* as you move your shoulders up and back, broadening across your chest as you draw your shoulder blades together. • *Exhale* as you move your shoulders down and forward, broadening across your upper back while contracting your chest.	Repeat for 10 breaths.
Bonus #8	**Neck Rotation**	*Do this exercise slowly. If this movement causes pain at any time, stop immediately.* • Look straight ahead. Keep your shoulders square in front of you. • *Inhale* and slowly turn your head to the **right**. • *Exhale* and slowly turn your head to the **left**.	Repeat for 5 breaths.
Bonus #9 Right Side	**Neck Side Stretch – Right Side**	*Do this exercise slowly. If this movement causes pain at any time, stop immediately.* • Bend your **right** arm at a right angle at your side with the **right** palm facing up, keeping your elbow close to your torso. • Place your **left** hand on the top of your head and slowly tilt your **left** ear toward your **left** shoulder. • Slowly apply gentle pressure with your **left** hand to increase the stretch.	Hold for 5 breaths.

Bonus #9 Left Side	**Neck Side Stretch– Left Side**	• Bend your **left** arm at a right angle at your side with the **left** palm facing up, keeping your elbow close to your torso. • Place your **right** hand on the top of your head and slowly tilt your **right** ear toward your **right** shoulder. • Apply gentle pressure with your **right** hand to increase the stretch.	Hold for 5 breaths.
Bonus #10	**Seated Leg Raises**	• Sit so that your low back touches the back of the chair. • Press your palms down on either side of your legs. • *Inhale* and stretch your legs out in front of you, as you pull your abdomen in. • Keeping your abdomen in and your core braced in this position, *exhale* and lift both of your legs as high as you comfortably can. • *Inhale* as you lower your legs, keeping your abdomen braced, pulling in.	Perform for 10 breaths.
Bonus #11	**Seated Meditation**	• Place your palms face up on your thighs. • Look straight ahead and close your eyes. • Picture in your mind a relaxing, peaceful scene, such as a still lake. • Focus only on this image as you listen to your breath.	Perform for 10 breaths

ACKNOWLEDGMENTS

The authors would like to thank Lauren, Mac, Jennifer, Adam, Micheale, Dan, Tiffany, Carolyn, Barbara, Paul, Heidi, Haili, Daisy and Lilly for their advice, input and inspiration.

ABOUT THE AUTHORS

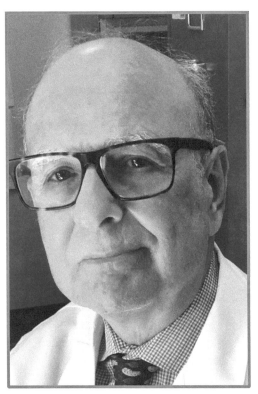

Walid M. Hafez, MD

Walid M. Hafez, MD, is a neurologist with over four decades of clinical experience. He has devoted his career to developing and providing comprehensive and compassionate care to patients with a broad range of neurological disorders. He has also lectured extensively on various topics, including MS, Parkinson's, epilepsy, and complications and treatment of headaches and strokes.

Dr. Hafez is board certified by the American Board of Electroencephalography and Neurophysiology Board, the American Board of Psychiatry and Neurology - Sleep Medicine Board, and the American Board of Psychiatry and Neurology – Neurology Board. He is also an FAA medical examiner.

Dr. Hafez is a graduate of the American University of Beirut Medical School in Beirut, Lebanon. He completed his neurology residency training at the University of Iowa College of Medicine. He was the Medical Director of the Blessing Hospital Rehabilitation Center from 1987 to 2009.

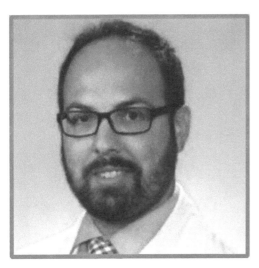

Zachary T. Hafez, MD

Zachary T. Hafez, MD, is an established and highly skilled physician in emergency medicine. He has published numerous articles on a wide range of topics, including cannabinoid hyperemesis syndrome and ultrasound enhanced thrombolysis.

Dr. Hafez is board certified in emergency medicine from the American Board of Emergency Medicine and is also board certified in Advanced Cardiac Life Support, Advanced Trauma Life Support, Basic Life Support and Pediatric Advanced Life Support. He is a graduate of the University of Missouri School of Medicine and completed his residency training at the Washington University School of Medicine. He holds an MS degree in bioengineering and BS degree in electrical engineering from the University of Illinois at Urbana-Champaign.

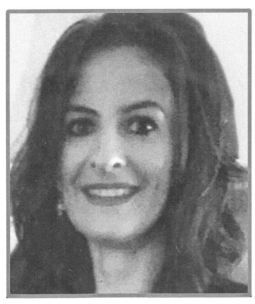

Amina M. Hafez

Amina M. Hafez is a certified yoga instructor and completed YogaWorks' 500-hour yoga teacher training program. She is also certified in barre by Exhale. Ms. Hafez has practiced yoga and pilates for over 15 years.

Ms. Hafez is also a lawyer and businesswoman and has worked in the fields of law and banking in New York and London for over 15 years. She graduated with a JD/MBA and BS in Accountancy from the University of Illinois at Urbana-Champaign. She was a Fulbright scholar in Germany.

CPSIA information can be obtained
at www.ICGtesting.com
Printed in the USA
BVHW020927130920
588612BV00004BA/23